The Surprisingly Useful

Health Logbook
Of Medical Care
Adult Version

**For Patients and Families to Facilitate
Communication and Shared Decisions**

This book belongs to ________________________________

Disclaimer. The contents of this log are intended to further understanding and encourage discussion only. This medical log is not intended and should not be relied upon as recommending or promoting a specific method, diagnosis or treatment. The publisher and the author make no representations or warranties with respect to the accuracy or completeness of the contents and specifically disclaim all warranties, including without limitation any implied warranties of fitness for a particular purpose. In view of ongoing research, equipment modifications, changes in government regulations, and the constant flow of information regarding the use of medicines, equipment and devices, the reader is urged to review and evaluate the information provided for each medicine, piece of equipment or device. The purpose of this book is to enhance and encourage discussion between each patient and their individual physician, not to replace in any way the information and instruction obtained through that dialogue. The fact that an organization or web site is referred to in this work as a potential source does not mean that the author or publisher endorses the information, organization or web site.

Table of Contents

What is the Point of a Medical Log?

This book came to me in one of those Zen moments. Years of experience, ideas about what is right and wrong about the doctor-patient relationship, and concerns about medical information were narrowed down to a single focus of insight and possible solution.

Here is what happened. I was going to see an elderly lady who was a patient in the hospital. She only spoke Russian. Next to the bed was a cheap spiral notebook. Her son had put it there and left a message on the top. *"Please read. Write down if you are going to change anything or order any tests so I can explain to my mom."* Because he could not be there during the day when the doctors made their rounds, he had devised a system of translation and communication. Every evening when he would visit her, he would write down his own concerns and those expressed to him by his mother. Then during the day the doctors and nurses could give answers to the questions. And hopefully write down what was going to happen. Then he would translate it all the next night when he got off work. But what I realized, in that moment when I looked at that notebook was that sons and daughters, husbands and wives, friends – all sorts of people - translated all of the time. In fact, patients filter and translate themselves at nearly every visit. They take medical speak and turn it into the language of "what does it mean to me?" There is the hurry of the doctor trying to care for many. There is the difficulty of the patient, trying to remember, trying to make sense of what they feel inside. Even patients who speak the same language as the doctor struggle. They want to be part of the process. They want to make themselves understood. Patients want to know where things are headed.

It was that moment for me, seeing the old tattered spiral bound notebook, probably co-opted from one of the grandkids; that is when I really saw that there was a solution. And for the first time in years, I realized there was a problem that we were not addressing. From our side, the doctor's side of the equation, we have become so used to less-than-optimal communication that we don't see it anymore. We are accustomed to medical information being unorganized. And we expect people to feel out of control. The solution that the spiral notebook offered was for a problem that had long been the standard of care.

So I read the notes my patient's son had made in the notebook. And then I took a moment to write a message back, about how we were going to repeat one of the tests and continue the same medications. And ever since then, I have seen everything in a different way.

Every single day, I see patients struggle over and over again. I see people attempt to keep track of their important medical information without having a tool for doing it. For years, I have watched people arrive with their information on scraps of paper, Post-its, the margins of prescriptions, the back of envelopes, napkins, and sometimes even blood pressures penned with ink on their palm. They struggle to remember the questions they wanted to ask and worry about the concerns they are sure they have forgotten. Patients tell me and studies confirm that even the most compliant patients often forget to complete what was requested of them. They forget some of the instructions. They choose to do something different because they do not understand the motivation or logic behind the decisions that were made by the doctor.

After that first discovery, the need for translation, for control, I realized it is our fault. We doctors have gotten exactly what we created. It might not be the outcome we intended, but the processes that we put in place made it inevitable. What I came to see is that it is going to take a change of philosophy. Creating this log has become more about changing the way people, both on the medical side and on the patient side view their roles. It is not that people are unable to handle their information and decision-making. The problem is that we have conditioned them otherwise. Somewhere in this last century we've taken away their right to be in control.

Consider the encounter I had in my office. There was a 42-year-old woman who was my patient. Her husband came to the visit with her. When I walked into the room, she was working on her grocery-shopping list. I could see there were all kinds of details about what type of cereal that each kid liked to eat, specific brands of hot dogs, and certain kinds of soup. There were certain snacks for the slumber party this coming weekend and other snacks for the Monday night football game. She also was running her electronic organizer. She had it turned on because she was supposed to bring a dessert to her nephew's birthday party. There was further information about the present that she was going to get him. He wanted a CD by a band she had never heard of and a gift certificate to a skateboard shop. The husband meanwhile was flipping through a Consumer Reports magazine. He was studying about home theatre surround sound systems. And there was a bookmark in another section about car tires that he wanted to review later because he was going to need new tires this next summer before they went on vacation.

"Hi." I shook their hands. "How's your blood pressure been?" I said to my patient. "You've been checking it, right. Got some numbers for me?" We had changed medications at her last visit.

"Oh…" she stammered. "Well, I didn't really get the cuff because the pharmacy had a couple of different kinds of machines. We weren't sure which would be best."

The husband looked from his wife to me and shrugged.

"Well," I continued, already feeling a bit defeated because we were going to have to guess without all of the information. "It looks better today than last time, but still not perfect. Did you start taking two of the bisoprolol?"

"I think we changed from the yellow to the red one. Isn't that right? But I only took one. That's what the prescription said on the bottle."

The husband listened, nodded his head, and then shrugged his shoulders in a sign of surrender.

"Well, yeah, it did say just one. That is all that the insurance will pay for. They won't let you have two a day.

We'll have to increase the strength. Remember, we talked about it though, how you'd go up to two if one wasn't working and then we could give the right dose at this visit." I flipped pages in the chart, reviewing my last note again to confirm that is what I told her. "So… I guess you are going to need to go up. It's high today. Maybe we should have you start taking two now. I hate to do that though, without really knowing where you have been running at home. But with this one number we have here in the office, it is still too high."

"That's because she forgot to take the pill this morning," the husband suddenly interjected, looking a bit guilty. "I usually put them out with my cholesterol stuff, but this morning I was running late and… well. I just forgot our pills."

"Oh that's right. He forgets pretty much every weekend. Or like this morning, we were going to come here so had breakfast together on the way." She sat up. "Do you think it would matter if I forgot to take the pill?"

I sighed.

Then I wondered, why could she remember the details about shopping? There was the name of a band that she has never heard of, but she wrote it down and will search through their CDs at the store until she finds the right one. She stored and sorted particular details about the family's grocery needs. Those were complicated tasks, involving a lot of specific information. The name of the band and the details about the skateboard shop were both unusual and out of her ordinary experience. And yet, she would remember what she needed to remember. She wrote down the parts that she might forget. And she would learn about the items with which she was not familiar. Then there was the husband. He would study about stereo systems and car tires. Yet he was unable to help make a decision about the twenty-five dollar purchase of a blood pressure cuff. He was organized enough to plan for the summer vacation, but often missed life-saving medication. Why did they perform so well in other parts of their life, yet be negligent when it came to medical issues?

That's when I realized that creating a log was more than just putting words on paper. For a moment I thought if they had my dreamed-of logbook, it wouldn't make a difference anyway. But then again, it might. In order for patients to take ownership of their personal medical information, it would require a philosophical change. After all, there are logs and diaries about all kinds of peripheral health issues. There are weight loss logs, food and nutrition logs, alternative medicine diaries. There are an abundance of diaries and record-keeping systems for exercise. That's health related, isn't it? There are places to record the details of pregnancy. There are immunization records that mom's are supposed to keep safe somewhere. But those are all in a certain realm; relegated to those areas of health that doctors allowed people to track on their own.

Further, most patients are intelligent enough to remember and make important decisions regarding a range of complicated information like grocery lists, sports teams and celebrity gossip. As a society, we like to be involved. From television shows like American Idol to on-line gaming, the trend is to be involved and help decide what is going to happen to the world around us. Why then, when it comes to medications and doctor visits do so many people go blank?

We tend to blame our patients for not knowing. If you hung out in the ER or lunch room where doctors and nurses talk, you would hear stories about how patients are "bad." They don't know the names of medications they take. They can't remember what surgeries they've had or which specialist they saw or when. For their part, patients are often amazed (when they do get a glimpse of their chart) that medical records are incomplete, not coordinated from one office to the next, and contain wrong information. But back to all those "bad" patients. For as long as I have been a doctor, the buzz has been to create patient-centered care. But I think we only really mean that when it is convenient to us in the medical community. As soon as patients really start asking to be part of the decision-making process, we get annoyed. Don't believe me? See what happens when a patient calls in and requests an MRI because he hurt his knee over the weekend. Or tells the doctor she wants to take an antibiotic or a particular brand of cholesterol medication because she saw it advertised on television. And it is not just doctors who want to control the information and make the decisions. In the examples mentioned above, not only would the doctor be reluctant but also the patient's insurance would not want to pay. In fact, I would say the trend had moved away from patient-centered care and away from physician-directed care for that matter. The trend for the last few years has been toward bureaucratic-dictated health care. Insurance companies increasingly tell all of us, what we can prescribe and when it is acceptable to order a test. But even that, I believe, can be helped by having an informed group of patients who are actively recording and understanding what is happening to them and helping make decisions.

Now I turn back to this book. When I decided that I was going to make a book for people to keep track of their medical information, I looked around for examples of what it should be. There are manuals for everything. From toys to televisions - everything has instructions. But that is not what I wanted. I needed something more along the lines of a diary. But not just someplace to record what happened after the fact. I want to give people a tool, to carry with them as they age. I believe people should be recording important information, sure. But I also wanted people to be more prepared, to use this book to get ready for what was going to happen. When I thought of the process of going to the doctor, of having a major illness or spending time in the hospital, I decided it was most like taking a trip. Living through our life is a journey. There are both predictable destinations and uncharted diversions. And when we travel, we tend to get prepared. We look at a map. We decide what language is spoken at our destination. We budget time and money. We ask questions. And people who travel a lot tend to keep logs. The most informed adventurers keep track of what you liked and did not like about a place, which restaurants were especially good and which hotels had

the best beds. So that is where I finally turned for the closest
example. Of course, I hope this book is really a combination
of all of those things: a diary, a log, a map, and a place to
prepare.

I entered practice 13 years ago. In that time, so much has
remained the same, such as the importance of listening and in
even many basic treatments. Antibiotics for infections, how to
control the risk factors for cardiovascular disease, and early
detection of cancer to prevent death and morbidity are nearly
the same now as when I started. But there have been some
bad changes. The number of patients that need to be cared
for by any given physician has increased. And there have
been good changes such as the ability to monitor blood
sugars, utilize nebulizer machines, and do heart
cathertizations and laproscopic surgeries. But one of the
biggest shifts in medicine has been the democratization of
medical information. In just a few decades, techniques and
methods of treatment went from proprietary, owned by a
single physician or group, to being available to others through
peer-reviewed publications. And in the last decade, that
information has become available to the public in part through
the Internet. It is perfectly possible that a patient might know
more about a certain topic of their interest than their
physician. There is nothing to stop anyone from learning. I
am optimistic that this book, your new Health Logbook, is part
of that trend. It is another step. I don't think an individual's
medical information has to be the property of a doctor or
hospital, hidden away in a chart that only certain people can
access. I don't think that a patient who is getting ready to
interact with the medical system needs to walk in unprepared.
I think everyone has the right to own, and should have full
permission to participate in, their health decisions.

My patient needed her son to translate how she felt, write
down the questions that she needed answered, and explain in
a language she could understand what was going to happen
to her. She and her son opened my eyes to the need for this

10

tool. I know that they taught me to be a better doctor. I hope
this book helps you be a better patient.

Personal History

Insurance and Number_____________________________

My primary care doctor ___________________________

Their phone number is ___________________________

<u>Specialist's name</u>   <u>phone number</u>

____

____

____

____

____

____

Who else can access your records? (HIPPA)
____

Do you have a living will? _________________________

Would you want artificial life support? _____________

Do you want CPR is your heart stops? _____________

Major/Chronic Illnesses (date of onset and doctors)

____

____

____

____

____

____

____

____

Surgeries/Pregnancies/Hospital (year and doctor)

____

____

____

____

____

____

____

____

Tobacco? ___________________________

Alcohol? ___________________________

Other drugs? _________________________

Family History (major illnesses):

Mother/Father ____________________________________

Siblings____

Other ____

Physicals, Tests and Immunizations

Routine (physicals, lab, Pap, mammo, colonoscopy)
Procedure   Date   Findings

____

____

____

____

____

____

____

____

Procedures or Tests (include radiology tests, etc.)
Test/Doctor   Reason   Outcome
        Date

____

____

____

____

____

____

____

Adult Immunizations   Completed Date

____

____

____

____

This would be a good place to keep track of cholesterol, PSA, etc.

Date   Test   Value

____

____

____

____

____

____

____

____

____

____

____

____

____

____

____

____

____

____

____

Vitals Tracking

This would be a good place to track weight, blood pressure, etc.

Date   Test   Value

____

____

____

____

____

____

____

____

____

____

____

____

____

____

____

____

____

____

____

____

____

____

Date	Test	Value

Medications

Date _______________

Drug Allergies ____

Pharmacy/Phone Number ______________________________

Medicine   Strength How Often Diagnosis Started

____

____

____

____

____

____

____

____

____

____

____

____

____

____

____

____

____

____

____

Date _________________

Drug Allergies _________________________________

Pharmacy/Phone Number _______________________________

Medicine   Strength How Often Diagnosis Started

____

____

____

____

____

____

____

____

____

____

____

____

____

____

____

____

____

____

____

____

____

____

____

____

Medications

Date _______________

Drug Allergies ____

Pharmacy/Phone Number _________________________________

Medicine   Strength How Often Diagnosis Started

____

____

____

____

____

____

____

____

____

____

____

____

____

____

____

____

____

____

____

____

____

____

Date _______________

Drug Allergies ____

Pharmacy/Phone Number ___________________________________

Medicine   Strength How Often Diagnosis Started

____

____

____

____

____

____

____

____

____

____

____

____

____

____

____

____

____

____

____

____

____

____

How to Use the Visit Pages

There is no wrong way to use this book. If you find it helpful in your healthcare, then it is accomplishing its purpose. I have structured the visit pages to reflect the information I think is important. It is my hope that by using the forms and following the advice in this book, each visit will be more efficient.

Symptoms. The patient should complete this section before the visit.
- If you are going in with a new complaint, write down the details: Is there pain? How often? How severe? What makes your symptom happen? What makes it stop? Is there anything that you tried already? What do you think was the cause?
- If the visit is a follow-up on a medication, record how the medication made you feel. Did it work? Were there side effects?
- If you can't be at the visit with the patient, record your concerns here.

What do I want to accomplish? I believe one of the biggest areas of miscommunication between patients and their doctors occurs around this question. And yet, it is a question that is often overlooked. Patients and their doctors have been trained to focus on symptoms. Medical training teaches us to be "objective", distant, without opinion. And while an objective approach is important in diagnosing and curing an illness, no encounter can be or should be without the opinion of the patient. The symptoms are always in the context of the patient's personal experience and concerns.

To illustrate I would like to give a common example of a symptom that has been well studied. When a patient comes into the office with the complaint of back pain, a large majority is worried that their pain could ultimately result in paralysis. Patients worry about losing function. They worry about loosing independence. Doctors on the other hand, know that back pain rarely results in anything so morbid. Most back pain is self-limited and goes away without ever causing harm.

We move quickly through the assessment, judging whether there is neurologic impact and danger. If we are not suspicious then within a couple of minutes are already considering treatment options, such as medication or physical therapy. So here is where that disconnect can occur. If the patient never says, "I am worried that I might become paralyzed," it is unlikely that the doctor will volunteer an opinion on that possibility. The doctor will probably not say, "I am not worried about you becoming paralyzed." It is not because we do not care. It is because we take the knowledge for granted. I have seen many patients leave a doctor's visit with the assumption that the doctor did not care, because they did not address their most important concern.

A whole book could be written regarding the subject of miscommunication between patients and doctors. But because this is an organizer and not a book, I have listed a few examples to prompt your own planning:

- Do you think my symptom means I have cancer?
- Am I going to be disabled? In other words, do you think I might not be able to use my arm, leg, brain, etc.?
- Am I going to become disfigured?
- I don't want to know the fancy medical term of what is wrong. All I really want is to know how do I get back to normal?
- Are there other people who have the same thing that I have?
- How do other patients cope with this problem?
- How long am I going to have pain?
- Am I going to look, act, or appear different?
- Is there something I did to make this happen?
- How do I make sure this does not happen again?
- Where can I learn more about this condition?

Again, this is a short list. And even if asked, there are many questions to which we do not have the answer. Sometimes it is hard for us to admit we don't know. At other times it is difficult for patients to accept that there is no answer. But at least if you define your concerns, the doctor can answer the right question.

One final comment regarding your doctor's visit concerns time. A frustrating issue for patients and their doctors is when a patient expects to accomplish more things than are possible in the time allowed. If a patient brings a long list of questions, and expects the doctor to discuss all of their concerns in a short amount of time, it not only strains the relationship but also is potentially dangerous. I encourage people to try to manage only a few concerns in a single visit. The average visit is about fifteen minutes. If each topic takes a few minutes to describe, examine, and plan treatment; it is obviously unrealistic to plan to fix ten things. An alternative is to schedule a longer visit. Many doctors, myself included, practice under a term called "advanced access". We attempt to not create follow-up visits unless absolutely necessary. We try to address as many things as possible at once, and not put those lists off until a future visit. But we would like to have the right amount of time to get everything done. So if you feel the questions you would like addressed are complex, or if your list is longer than normal, let the office know ahead of time. Ask to schedule a longer visit. That is the courteous thing to do for other patients. It is also safer for you, so that the doctor can devote the proper amount of time needed to discuss your problem.

Response from doctor. The doctor or nurse might want to write down in their own words what they are thinking or advising. Or office personnel could fill in information about the follow-up tests or visits. If not, take a moment during or immediately afterward to record what was discussed. The sooner it is written down, the better. The conversation will still be fresh and probably more accurate. Then you can refer to this later, or share it with people who are trying to help with health decisions. It might even be that there are times when one doctor would like to use your log to see what another doctor said.

Tests ordered. This is pretty self-explanatory. But again, it might be good to ask what is the goal of the test or therapy. What does the doctor expect to accomplish with the referral?

I am surprised how often people go somewhere, or do something without actually knowing why.

Medication changes. Stopping a medication is just as important as starting a therapy. Even if you are just changing the dose, it should be recorded.

Follow-up. Every single encounter with your physician has some follow-up. Even if no visit is scheduled, doctors usually say, "as needed". Ask what that means. What are a few specific criteria that would indicate a need for a follow-up visit? Is it a particular number on the blood pressure readings? Or a certain number of days that should pass before you know you are not getting better? Ask for the important details and put them down on paper so you can refer to them later.

Finally, and again, this is your book. The purpose is to give you control over the information so you can ask the right questions and make informed decisions. I know a few doctors who still think all of the information, and decision-making, should be left to them. They might not like the idea of patients participating in the management of their own data. However, I think this would be rare. In my own practice, and knowing how my partners and the specialists to whom I refer practice medicine, I think we are eager to get the important information in the most efficient way. If your doctor seems uneasy, reassure them that you are only trying to consolidating those scraps of paper, organizing the thoughts in your head, and trying to make the best use of everyone's time.

Date ______________________________

Doctor ______________________________

Symptoms. Response to therapy.

____
____
____
____
____
____
____
____
____

What do I want to accomplish?

____
____
____
____
____
____
____
____
____

Never be afraid to try something new. Remember that a lone amateur built the Ark. A large group of professionals built the Titanic.   — Dave Barry

Response from doctor.

____
____
____
____
____
____
____
____
____
____

Tests ordered or referrals to other doctors, therapies.
(who schedules? time/place)

____
____
____

Medication changes. (starts, stops, dose changes)

____
____
____

Follow-up. (scheduled? or as needed? In person,
phone, mail?)

____
____
____
____
____

Date ___________________________________

Doctor ___________________________________

Symptoms. Response to therapy.

____
____
____
____
____
____
____
____
____

What do I want to accomplish?

____
____
____
____
____
____
____
____
____

Gardens are not made by sitting in the shade.
— Rudyard Kipling

Response from doctor.

Tests ordered or referrals to other doctors, therapies. (Who schedules? time/place)

Medication changes. (starts, stops, dose changes)

Follow-up. (scheduled? or as needed? In person, phone, mail?)

Date _______________________________________

Doctor _______________________________________

Symptoms. Response to therapy.

____
____
____
____
____
____
____
____

What do I want to accomplish?

____
____
____
____
____
____
____
____
____

A great secret of success is to go through life as a man who never gets used up.   — Albert Schweitzer

Response from doctor.

____
____
____
____
____
____
____
____
____
____

Tests ordered or referrals to other doctors, therapies.
(Who schedules? time/place)

____
____
____

Medication changes. (starts, stops, dose changes)

____
____
____

Follow-up. (scheduled? or as needed? In person,
phone, mail?)

____
____
____
____
____

Date _______________________________

Doctor _______________________________

Symptoms. Response to therapy.

What do I want to accomplish?

You can only perceive real beauty in a person as they get older.   – Anouk Aimee

Response from doctor.

____

____

____

____

____

____

____

____

____

Tests ordered or referrals to other doctors, therapies.
(Who schedules? time/place)

____

____

____

Medication changes. (starts, stops, dose changes)

____

____

____

Follow-up. (scheduled? or as needed? In person,
phone, mail?)

____

____

____

Date ___________________________________

Doctor _________________________________

Symptoms. Response to therapy.

____

____

____

____

____

____

____

____

What do I want to accomplish?

____

____

____

____

____

____

____

____

____

*How we spend our days is, of course, how we spend
our lives.*   *– Anne Dillard*

Response from doctor.

____
____
____
____
____
____
____
____
____
____

Tests ordered or referrals to other doctors, therapies.
(Who schedules? time/place)

____
____
____
____

Medication changes. (starts, stops, dose changes)

____
____
____

Follow-up. (scheduled? or as needed? In person,
phone, mail?)

____
____
____
____

Date ___________________________________

Doctor ___________________________________

Symptoms. Response to therapy.

____

____
____
____
____
____
____
____
____

What do I want to accomplish?

____
____
____
____
____
____
____
____

Life is not a journey to the grave with the intention of arriving safely in a pretty and well-preserved body. But rather, to skid in broadside, thoroughly used up, totally worn out and proclaiming… "Wow, what a ride!!!"
- Unknown

Response from doctor.

____
____
____
____
____
____
____
____
____

Tests ordered or referrals to other doctors, therapies.
(Who schedules? time/place)

____
____
____

Medication changes. (starts, stops, dose changes)

____
____
____

Follow-up. (scheduled? or as needed? In person,
phone, mail?)

____
____
____
____

Date _________________________________

Doctor _________________________________

Symptoms. Response to therapy.

____
____
____
____
____
____
____
____

What do I want to accomplish?

____
____
____
____
____
____
____
____

Love is staying up all night with a sick child – or a healthy adult.   *– Sir David Paradine Frost*

Response from doctor.

Tests ordered or referrals to other doctors, therapies. (Who schedules? time/place)

Medication changes. (starts, stops, dose changes)

Follow-up. (scheduled? or as needed? In person, phone, mail?)

Date _______________________________

Doctor _______________________________

Symptoms. Response to therapy.

____
____
____
____
____
____
____
____

What do I want to accomplish?

____
____
____
____
____
____
____
____
____
____

It is part of the cure to wish to be cured.
– Alexander Pope

Response from doctor.

____
____
____
____
____
____
____
____
____
____

Tests ordered or referrals to other doctors, therapies.
(Who schedules? time/place)

____
____
____
____

Medication changes. (starts, stops, dose changes)

____
____
____
____

Follow-up. (scheduled? or as needed? In person,
phone, mail?)

____
____
____
____

Date _______________________________

Doctor _______________________________

Symptoms. Response to therapy.

____
____
____
____
____
____
____
____

What do I want to accomplish?

____
____
____
____
____
____
____
____

Life is a progress, and not a station.
                                    — Ralph Waldo Emerson

Response from doctor.

Tests ordered or referrals to other doctors, therapies. (Who schedules? time/place)

Medication changes. (starts, stops, dose changes)

Follow-up. (scheduled? or as needed? In person, phone, mail?)

Date _______________________________

Doctor _______________________________

Symptoms. Response to therapy.

____

____

____

____

____

____

____

____

What do I want to accomplish?

____

____

____

____

____

____

____

____

____

____

Love cures people – both the ones who give it and the ones who receive it. – Dr. Karl Menninger

Response from doctor.

____
____
____
____
____
____
____
____
____
____

Tests ordered or referrals to other doctors, therapies.
(Who schedules? time/place)

____
____
____
____

Medication changes. (starts, stops, dose changes)

____
____
____
____

Follow-up. (scheduled? or as needed? In person,
phone, mail?)

____
____
____
____

Date ________________________________

Doctor ________________________________

Symptoms. Response to therapy.

____
____
____
____
____
____
____
____

What do I want to accomplish?

____
____
____
____
____
____
____
____
____
____

A sailor without a destination cannot hope for a favorable wind.
                                        — Leon Tec

Response from doctor.

____
____
____
____
____
____
____
____
____
____
____

Tests ordered or referrals to other doctors, therapies. (Who schedules? time/place)

____
____
____
____

Medication changes. (starts, stops, dose changes)

____
____
____
____

Follow-up. (scheduled? or as needed? In person, phone, mail?)

____
____
____
____

Date _________________________________

Doctor _______________________________

Symptoms. Response to therapy.

____
____
____
____
____
____
____
____

What do I want to accomplish?

____
____
____
____
____
____
____
____

The optimism of a healthy mind is indefatigable.
— Margery Allingham

Response from doctor.

____
____
____
____
____
____
____
____
____
____

Tests ordered or referrals to other doctors, therapies.
(Who schedules? time/place)

____
____
____
____

Medication changes. (starts, stops, dose changes)

____
____
____

Follow-up. (scheduled? or as needed? In person,
phone, mail?)

____
____
____
____

Date _______________________________

Doctor _______________________________

Symptoms. Response to therapy.

____
____
____
____
____
____
____
____
____

What do I want to accomplish?

____
____
____
____
____
____
____
____
____
____

Habits are safer than rules; you don't have to watch them. And you don't have to keep them either; they keep you. – Dr. Frank Crane

Response from doctor.

____

____

____

____

____

____

____

____

____

____

Tests ordered or referrals to other doctors, therapies.
(Who schedules? time/place)

____

____

____

____

Medication changes. (starts, stops, dose changes)

____

____

____

____

Follow-up. (scheduled? or as needed? In person,
phone, mail?)

____

____

____

____

Date ________________________________

Doctor ________________________________

Symptoms. Response to therapy.

____
____
____
____
____
____
____
____
____

What do I want to accomplish?

____
____
____
____
____
____
____
____
____
____

A family is a unit composed not only of children but of men, women, an occasional animal, and the common cold.
— Ogden Nash

Response from doctor.

____
____
____
____
____
____
____
____
____
____

Tests ordered or referrals to other doctors, therapies.
(Who schedules? time/place)

____
____
____
____

Medication changes. (starts, stops, dose changes)

____
____
____
____

Follow-up. (scheduled? or as needed? In person,
phone, mail?)

____
____
____
____

Date _______________________________

Doctor _______________________________

Symptoms. Response to therapy.

____

What do I want to accomplish?

____

Old age is the most unexpected of all the things that can happen to a man. — James Thurber

Response from doctor.

Tests ordered or referrals to other doctors, therapies.
(Who schedules? time/place)

Medication changes. (starts, stops, dose changes)

Follow-up. (scheduled? or as needed? In person,
phone, mail?)

Date ___________________________________

Doctor _________________________________

Symptoms. Response to therapy.

____

____

____

____

____

____

____

____

What do I want to accomplish?

____

____

____

____

____

____

____

____

Hope begins in the dark, the stubborn hope that if you just show up and try to do the right thing, the dawn will come. You wait and watch and work: You don't give up. — Anne Lamott

Response from doctor.

____

____

____

____

____

____

____

____

____

____

Tests ordered or referrals to other doctors, therapies.
(Who schedules? time/place)

____

____

____

____

Medication changes. (starts, stops, dose changes)

____

____

____

____

Follow-up. (scheduled? or as needed? In person,
phone, mail?)

____

____

____

____

Date ________________________________

Doctor ________________________________

Symptoms. Response to therapy.

____
____
____
____
____
____
____
____

What do I want to accomplish?

____
____
____
____
____
____
____
____

Life ultimately means taking the responsibility to find the right answer to its problems and to fulfill the tasks which it constantly sets for each individual.
— Victor Frankl

Response from doctor.

____

____

____

____

____

____

____

____

____

____

Tests ordered or referrals to other doctors, therapies.
(Who schedules? time/place)

____

____

____

____

Medication changes. (starts, stops, dose changes)

____

____

____

Follow-up. (scheduled? or as needed? In person,
phone, mail?)

____

____

____

____

Date ______________________________

Doctor ______________________________

Symptoms. Response to therapy.

____
____
____
____
____
____
____
____

What do I want to accomplish?

____
____
____
____
____
____
____
____
____

*Treasure the love you receive above all. It will
survive long after your good health has vanished.*
— Og Mandino

Response from doctor.

____
____
____
____
____
____
____
____

Tests ordered or referrals to other doctors, therapies.
(Who schedules? time/place)

____
____
____
____

Medication changes. (starts, stops, dose changes)

____
____
____
____

Follow-up. (scheduled? or as needed? In person,
phone, mail?)

____
____
____
____

Date _______________________________

Doctor _____________________________

Symptoms. Response to therapy.

____
____
____
____
____
____
____
____
____

What do I want to accomplish?

____
____
____
____
____
____
____
____
____

Our body is a machine for living. It is organized for that, it is nature. Let life go on in it unhindered and let it defend itself, it will do more than if you paralyze it with remedies.
— Leo Tolstoy

Response from doctor.

____

____

____

____

____

____

____

____

____

Tests ordered or referrals to other doctors, therapies.
(Who schedules? time/place)

____

____

____

____

Medication changes. (starts, stops, dose changes)

____

____

____

____

Follow-up. (scheduled? or as needed? In person,
phone, mail?)

____

____

____

____

Date _______________________________

Doctor _______________________________

Symptoms. Response to therapy.

____
____
____
____
____
____
____
____

What do I want to accomplish?

____
____
____
____
____
____
____
____
____
____

The only way to keep your health is to eat what you don't want, drink what you don't like, and do what you'd rather not.
— Mark Twain

Response from doctor.

____

____

____

____

____

____

____

____

____

Tests ordered or referrals to other doctors, therapies.
(Who schedules? time/place)

____

____

____

____

Medication changes. (starts, stops, dose changes)

____

____

____

____

Follow-up. (scheduled? or as needed? In person,
phone, mail?)

____

____

____

____

Date ____________________________________

Doctor ________________________________

Symptoms. Response to therapy.

____
____
____
____
____
____
____
____
____

What do I want to accomplish?

____
____
____
____
____
____
____
____
____
____
____

Old people shouldn't eat health foods. They need all the preservatives they can get.   – Robert Orben

Response from doctor.

Tests ordered or referrals to other doctors, therapies. (Who schedules? time/place)

Medication changes. (starts, stops, dose changes)

Follow-up. (scheduled? or as needed? In person, phone, mail?)

Date ___________________________________

Doctor _________________________________

Symptoms. Response to therapy.

____
____
____
____
____
____
____
____
____

What do I want to accomplish?

____
____
____
____
____
____
____
____
____

God heals, and the doctor takes the fees.
                              – Benjamin Franklin

Response from doctor.

____

____

____

____

____

____

____

____

____

Tests ordered or referrals to other doctors, therapies.
(Who schedules? time/place)

____

____

____

____

Medication changes. (starts, stops, dose changes)

____

____

____

____

Follow-up. (scheduled? or as needed? In person,
phone, mail?)

____

____

____

____

Date __________________________________

Doctor _______________________________

Symptoms. Response to therapy.

____

What do I want to accomplish?

____

Cheerfulness, sir, is the principle ingredient in the composition of health. — Arthur Murphy

Response from doctor.

____

____

____

____

____

____

____

____

____

Tests ordered or referrals to other doctors, therapies.
(Who schedules? time/place)

____

____

____

____

Medication changes. (starts, stops, dose changes)

____

____

____

____

Follow-up. (scheduled? or as needed? In person,
phone, mail?)

____

____

____

____

____

Date _______________________________

Doctor _______________________________

Symptoms. Response to therapy.

____
____
____
____
____
____
____
____

What do I want to accomplish?

____
____
____
____
____
____
____
____
____

To me, old age is always 15 years older than I am.
– Bernard Baruch

Response from doctor.

____
____
____
____
____
____
____
____
____

Tests ordered or referrals to other doctors, therapies.
(Who schedules? time/place)

____
____
____
____

Medication changes. (starts, stops, dose changes)

____
____
____
____

Follow-up. (scheduled? or as needed? In person,
phone, mail?)

____
____
____
____

Date _______________________________

Doctor _______________________________

Symptoms. Response to therapy.

____
____
____
____
____
____
____
____

What do I want to accomplish?

____
____
____
____
____
____
____
____
____
____

All would live long, but none would be old.
— Benjamin Franklin

Response from doctor.

Tests ordered or referrals to other doctors, therapies. (Who schedules? time/place)

Medication changes. (starts, stops, dose changes)

Follow-up. (scheduled? or as needed? In person, phone, mail?)

Date ____________________________

Doctor ____________________________

Symptoms. Response to therapy.

What do I want to accomplish?

You don't stop laughing because you grow old. You grow old because you stop laughing.

— Michael Pritchard

Response from doctor.

____
____
____
____
____
____
____
____
____
____

Tests ordered or referrals to other doctors, therapies. (Who schedules? time/place)

____
____
____
____

Medication changes. (starts, stops, dose changes)

____
____
____
____

Follow-up. (scheduled? or as needed? In person, phone, mail?)

____
____
____
____

Date _______________________________

Doctor _______________________________

Symptoms. Response to therapy.

____
____
____
____
____
____
____
____

What do I want to accomplish?

____
____
____
____
____
____
____
____
____
____
____

Life isn't fair. It's just fairer than death, that's all.
— William Goldman

Response from doctor.

____

____

____

____

____

____

____

____

____

Tests ordered or referrals to other doctors, therapies.
(Who schedules? time/place)

____

____

____

____

Medication changes. (starts, stops, dose changes)

____

____

____

____

Follow-up. (scheduled? or as needed? In person,
phone, mail?)

____

____

____

____

Date _______________________________

Doctor ____________________________

Symptoms. Response to therapy.

What do I want to accomplish?

The longer I live the more beautiful life becomes.
— Frank Lloyd Wright

Response from doctor.

____

____

____

____

____

____

____

____

____

Tests ordered or referrals to other doctors, therapies.
(Who schedules? time/place)

____

____

____

____

Medication changes. (starts, stops, dose changes)

____

____

____

____

Follow-up. (scheduled? or as needed? In person,
phone, mail?)

____

____

____

____

Date ___________________________________

Doctor _________________________________

Symptoms. Response to therapy.

____
____
____
____
____
____
____
____

What do I want to accomplish?

____
____
____
____
____
____
____
____

The healthy, the strong individual, is the one who asks for help when he needs it. Whether he has an abscess on his knee or in his soul. – Rona Barrett

Response from doctor.

____

____

____

____

____

____

____

____

____

Tests ordered or referrals to other doctors, therapies.
(Who schedules? time/place)

____

____

____

____

Medication changes. (starts, stops, dose changes)

____

____

____

____

Follow-up. (scheduled? or as needed? In person,
phone, mail?)

____

____

____

____

Date ___________________________________

Doctor _________________________________

Symptoms. Response to therapy.

____
____
____
____
____
____
____
____

What do I want to accomplish?

____
____
____
____
____
____
____
____
____
____

What some call health, if purchased by perpetual anxiety about diet, isn't much better than tedious disease. — George Dennison Prentice

84

Response from doctor.

____
____
____
____
____
____
____
____
____
____

Tests ordered or referrals to other doctors, therapies.
(Who schedules? time/place)

____
____
____
____

Medication changes. (starts, stops, dose changes)

____
____
____
____

Follow-up. (scheduled? or as needed? In person,
phone, mail?)

____
____
____
____

Date _______________________________________

Doctor _____________________________________

Symptoms. Response to therapy.

____

____

____

____

____

____

____

____

What do I want to accomplish?

____

____

____

____

____

____

____

____

Any healthy man can go without food for two days –
but not without poetry. — Charles Baudelaire

Response from doctor.

____

____

____

____

____

____

____

____

____

Tests ordered or referrals to other doctors, therapies.
(Who schedules? time/place)

____

____

____

____

Medication changes. (starts, stops, dose changes)

____

____

____

____

Follow-up. (scheduled? or as needed? In person,
phone, mail?)

____

____

____

____

Date _______________________________

Doctor _______________________________

Symptoms. Response to therapy.

____
____
____
____
____
____
____

What do I want to accomplish?

____
____
____
____
____
____
____

The secret of health for both mind and body is not to mourn for the past, worry about the future, or anticipate troubles but to live in the present moment wisely and earnestly. — Buddha

Response from doctor.

____
____
____
____
____
____
____
____
____

Tests ordered or referrals to other doctors, therapies.
(Who schedules? time/place)

____
____
____
____

Medication changes. (starts, stops, dose changes)

____
____
____
____

Follow-up. (scheduled? or as needed? In person,
phone, mail?)

____
____
____
____

Date ________________________________

Doctor ________________________________

Symptoms. Response to therapy.

____
____
____
____
____
____
____
____

What do I want to accomplish?

____
____
____
____
____
____
____
____
____
____

A man's health can be judged by which he takes two at a time – pills or stairs.
— Joan Welsh

Response from doctor.

____

____

____

____

____

____

____

____

____

____

Tests ordered or referrals to other doctors, therapies.
(Who schedules? time/place)

____

____

____

____

Medication changes. (starts, stops, dose changes)

____

____

____

____

Follow-up. (scheduled? or as needed? In person,
phone, mail?)

____

____

____

____

Date _________________________________

Doctor _______________________________

Symptoms. Response to therapy.

____
____
____
____
____
____
____
____
____

What do I want to accomplish?

____
____
____
____
____
____
____
____
____
____

Doctors don't know everything really. They understand matter, not spirit. And you and I live in spirit.
— William Saroyan

Response from doctor.

____

____

____

____

____

____

____

____

____

Tests ordered or referrals to other doctors, therapies.
(Who schedules? time/place)

____

____

____

____

Medication changes. (starts, stops, dose changes)

____

____

____

____

Follow-up. (scheduled? or as needed? In person,
phone, mail?)

____

____

____

____

Date ___________________________________

Doctor ___________________________________

Symptoms. Response to therapy.

____
____
____
____
____
____
____
____

What do I want to accomplish?

____
____
____
____
____
____
____
____
____
____

Every patient carries her or his own doctor inside.
– Albert Schweitzer

Response from doctor.

____
____
____
____
____
____
____
____
____
____

Tests ordered or referrals to other doctors, therapies.
(Who schedules? time/place)

____
____
____
____

Medication changes. (starts, stops, dose changes)

____
____
____
____

Follow-up. (scheduled? or as needed? In person,
phone, mail?)

____
____
____

Date _______________________________

Doctor _____________________________

Symptoms. Response to therapy.

____

____

____

____

____

____

____

What do I want to accomplish?

____

____

____

____

____

____

____

No man should go through life without once experiencing healthy, even bored solitude in the wilderness, finding himself depending solely on himself and thereby learning his true and hidden strength. — Jack Kerouac

Response from doctor.

____
____
____
____
____
____
____
____
____
____

Tests ordered or referrals to other doctors, therapies.
(Who schedules? time/place)

____
____
____
____

Medication changes. (starts, stops, dose changes)

____
____
____

Follow-up. (scheduled? or as needed? In person,
phone, mail?)

____
____
____

Date _______________________________

Doctor _______________________________

Symptoms. Response to therapy.

____
____
____
____
____
____
____
____

What do I want to accomplish?

____
____
____
____
____
____
____
____
____
____

It is better not to express what one means, than to express what one does not mean. — Karl Kraus

Response from doctor.

____

____

____

____

____

____

____

____

____

____

Tests ordered or referrals to other doctors, therapies.
(Who schedules? time/place)

____

____

____

Medication changes. (starts, stops, dose changes)

____

____

____

Follow-up. (scheduled? or as needed? In person,
phone, mail?)

____

____

____

____

Date ________________________________

Doctor __________________________________

Symptoms. Response to therapy.

____
____
____
____
____
____
____
____

What do I want to accomplish?

____
____
____
____
____
____
____
____

Health is not valued until sickness comes.
— Thomas Fuller

Response from doctor.

____
____
____
____
____
____
____
____
____
____

Tests ordered or referrals to other doctors, therapies.
(Who schedules? time/place)

____
____
____

Medication changes. (starts, stops, dose changes)

____
____
____

Follow-up. (scheduled? or as needed? In person,
phone, mail?)

____
____
____
____

Date _________________________________

Doctor _______________________________

Symptoms. Response to therapy.

____
____
____
____
____
____
____
____

What do I want to accomplish?

____
____
____
____
____
____
____
____

You can either hold yourself up to the unrealistic standards of others, or ignore them and concentrate on being happy with yourself as you are.

— Jeph Jacques

Response from doctor.

____
____
____
____
____
____
____
____
____
____

Tests ordered or referrals to other doctors, therapies.
(Who schedules? time/place)

____
____
____

Medication changes. (starts, stops, dose changes)

____
____
____

Follow-up. (scheduled? or as needed? In person,
phone, mail?)

____
____
____
____

Date _______________________________

Doctor _______________________________

Symptoms. Response to therapy.

____
____
____
____
____
____
____
____

What do I want to accomplish?

____
____
____
____
____
____
____
____

Be careful about reading health books. You may die of a misprint.
— Mark Twain

104

Response from doctor.

____
____
____
____
____
____
____
____
____
____

Tests ordered or referrals to other doctors, therapies.
(Who schedules? time/place)

____
____
____

Medication changes. (starts, stops, dose changes)

____
____
____

Follow-up. (scheduled? or as needed? In person,
phone, mail?)

____
____
____
____

Date ___________________________________

Doctor ___________________________________

Symptoms. Response to therapy.

____

____
____
____
____
____
____
____
____

What do I want to accomplish?

____
____
____
____
____
____
____
____
____

Of one thing I am certain, the body is not the measure of healing – peace is the measure.

– George Melton

Response from doctor.

Tests ordered or referrals to other doctors, therapies.
(Who schedules? time/place)

Medication changes. (starts, stops, dose changes)

Follow-up. (scheduled? or as needed? In person,
phone, mail?)

Date ___________________________________

Doctor _________________________________

Symptoms. Response to therapy.

____

____

____

____

____

____

____

____

What do I want to accomplish?

____

____

____

____

____

____

____

____

____

A sound mind in a sound body is a short but full description of a happy state in this world.

— John Locke

Response from doctor.

____
____
____
____
____
____
____
____
____
____

Tests ordered or referrals to other doctors, therapies.
(Who schedules? time/place)

____
____
____

Medication changes. (starts, stops, dose changes)

____
____
____

Follow-up. (scheduled? or as needed? In person,
phone, mail?)

____
____
____
____

Date _______________________________

Doctor _______________________________

Symptoms. Response to therapy.

____
____
____
____
____
____
____
____

What do I want to accomplish?

____
____
____
____
____
____
____
____
____

Hope is necessary in every condition.
                              – Samuel Johnson

Response from doctor.

____
____
____
____
____
____
____
____
____
____

Tests ordered or referrals to other doctors, therapies.
(Who schedules? time/place)

____
____
____

Medication changes. (starts, stops, dose changes)

____
____
____

Follow-up. (scheduled? or as needed? In person,
phone, mail?)

____
____
____

Date ___________________________________

Doctor ___________________________________

Symptoms. Response to therapy.

____
____
____
____
____
____
____
____

What do I want to accomplish?

____
____
____
____
____
____
____
____
____

The soul of man is immortal and imperishable

– Plato

Response from doctor.

Tests ordered or referrals to other doctors, therapies.
(Who schedules? time/place)

Medication changes. (starts, stops, dose changes)

Follow-up. (scheduled? or as needed? In person,
phone, mail?)

Date _______________________________

Doctor _______________________________

Symptoms. Response to therapy.

____
____
____
____
____
____
____
____

What do I want to accomplish?

____
____
____
____
____
____
____
____
____

Always laugh when you can. It is cheap medicine.
– Lord Byron

Response from doctor.

____
____
____
____
____
____
____
____
____
____

Tests ordered or referrals to other doctors, therapies.
(Who schedules? time/place)

____
____
____

Medication changes. (starts, stops, dose changes)

____
____
____

Follow-up. (scheduled? or as needed? In person,
phone, mail?)

____
____
____
____

Date _________________________________

Doctor _______________________________

Symptoms. Response to therapy.

____
____
____
____
____
____
____
____
____

What do I want to accomplish?

____
____
____
____
____
____
____
____
____
____

Science is organized knowledge. Wisdom is organized life.
                            – Immanuel Kant

Response from doctor.

____
____
____
____
____
____
____
____
____
____

Tests ordered or referrals to other doctors, therapies.
(Who schedules? time/place)

____
____
____

Medication changes. (starts, stops, dose changes)

____
____
____

Follow-up. (scheduled? or as needed? In person,
phone, mail?)

____
____
____
____

Date _______________________________

Doctor _______________________________

Symptoms. Response to therapy.

____
____
____
____
____
____
____
____

What do I want to accomplish?

____
____
____
____
____
____
____

I think a hero is an ordinary individual who finds strength to persevere and endure in spite of overwhelming obstacles. — Christopher Reeve

Response from doctor.

____
____
____
____
____
____
____
____
____
____

Tests ordered or referrals to other doctors, therapies.
(Who schedules? time/place)

____
____
____

Medication changes. (starts, stops, dose changes)

____
____
____

Follow-up. (scheduled? or as needed? In person,
phone, mail?)

____
____
____
____

Date ___________________________________

Doctor _________________________________

Symptoms. Response to therapy.

____
____
____
____
____
____
____
____

What do I want to accomplish?

____
____
____
____
____
____
____
____

Youth would be an ideal state if it came a little later in life.
— Herbert Henry Asquith

Response from doctor.

____

____

____

____

____

____

____

____

____

Tests ordered or referrals to other doctors, therapies.
(Who schedules? time/place)

____

____

____

Medication changes. (starts, stops, dose changes)

____

____

____

Follow-up. (scheduled? or as needed? In person,
phone, mail?)

____

____

____

____

Date ___________________________________

Doctor _________________________________

Symptoms. Response to therapy.

____
____
____
____
____
____
____
____

What do I want to accomplish?

____
____
____
____
____
____
____
____

Health can be squandered, but not stored up.
– Mason Cooley

Response from doctor.

____
____
____
____
____
____
____
____
____
____

Tests ordered or referrals to other doctors, therapies.
(Who schedules? time/place)

____
____
____

Medication changes. (starts, stops, dose changes)

____
____
____

Follow-up. (scheduled? or as needed? In person,
phone, mail?)

____
____
____

Date ___________________________________

Doctor _________________________________

Symptoms. Response to therapy.

____
____
____
____
____
____
____
____

What do I want to accomplish?

____
____
____
____
____
____
____
____
____

Health is my expected heaven.   – John Keats

Response from doctor.

____

____

____

____

____

____

____

____

____

Tests ordered or referrals to other doctors, therapies.
(Who schedules? time/place)

____

____

____

Medication changes. (starts, stops, dose changes)

____

____

____

Follow-up. (scheduled? or as needed? In person,
phone, mail?)

____

____

____

____

Date _________________________________

Doctor _______________________________

Symptoms. Response to therapy.

____
____
____
____
____
____
____
____
____

What do I want to accomplish?

____
____
____
____
____
____
____
____
____

There is more to life than increasing its speed.
                                    – Gandhi

Response from doctor.

____

____

____

____

____

____

____

____

____

____

Tests ordered or referrals to other doctors, therapies.
(Who schedules? time/place)

____

____

____

Medication changes. (starts, stops, dose changes)

____

____

____

Follow-up. (scheduled? or as needed? In person,
phone, mail?)

____

____

____

____

Date _______________________________

Doctor _______________________________

Symptoms. Response to therapy.

____
____
____
____
____
____
____
____

What do I want to accomplish?

____
____
____
____
____
____
____
____

We can not seek or attain health, wealth, learning, justice or kindness in general. Action is always specific, concrete, individualized, unique.

— Benjamin Jowett

Response from doctor.

____
____
____
____
____
____
____
____
____

Tests ordered or referrals to other doctors, therapies.
(Who schedules? time/place)

____
____
____

Medication changes. (starts, stops, dose changes)

____
____
____

Follow-up. (scheduled? or as needed? In person,
phone, mail?)

____
____
____
____

Date _______________________________

Doctor _______________________________

Symptoms. Response to therapy.

____

____
____
____
____
____
____
____
____

What do I want to accomplish?

____
____
____
____
____
____
____
____

Always bear in mind that your own resolution to succeed is more important than any other one thing.
— Abraham Lincoln

Response from doctor.

____
____
____
____
____
____
____
____
____

Tests ordered or referrals to other doctors, therapies.
(Who schedules? time/place)

____
____
____

Medication changes. (starts, stops, dose changes)

____
____
____

Follow-up. (scheduled? or as needed? In person,
phone, mail?)

____
____
____
____

Date _______________________________

Doctor _______________________________

Symptoms. Response to therapy.

____
____
____
____
____
____
____
____
____

What do I want to accomplish?

____
____
____
____
____
____
____
____
____

Health is not simply the absence of sickness.
— Hannah Green

Response from doctor.

Tests ordered or referrals to other doctors, therapies.
(Who schedules? time/place)

Medication changes. (starts, stops, dose changes)

Follow-up. (scheduled? or as needed? In person,
phone, mail?)

Date _______________________________

Doctor _____________________________

Symptoms. Response to therapy.

____
____
____
____
____
____
____
____

What do I want to accomplish?

____
____
____
____
____
____
____
____
____

Use it or loose it.   — Ralph Waldo Emerson

Response from doctor.

____
____
____
____
____
____
____
____
____
____

Tests ordered or referrals to other doctors, therapies.
(Who schedules? time/place)

____
____
____

Medication changes. (starts, stops, dose changes)

____
____
____

Follow-up. (scheduled? or as needed? In person,
phone, mail?)

____
____
____
____

Blood Tests

Complete Blood Count (CBC). A Complete Blood Count measures more than one thing and usually includes the number of white blood cells, which could reflect infection or problems with the bone marrow. The hemoglobin and hematocrit are ways of looking at the amount of red blood cells in our system. If the numbers are too low, then the patient is anemic.

Comprehensive Metabolic Panel (CMP) A Comprehensive Metabolic Panel measures around a dozen different items, including blood sugar, sodium, and potassium, liver function, and kidney function.

Lipid Panel. Lipid is a broad term for the group of tests relating to cholesterol.

- Total Cholesterol. This is the number usually meant when someone says "cholesterol."
- HDL. High Density Lipoprotein is the "good" cholesterol that scrubs out the arteries. Higher is better.
- LDL. Low Density Lipoprotein is the "bad" cholesterol that blocks up the arteries. The lower the better.
- Triglyceride is the third measurement. This measure of fat in our blood stream is the part that varies the most and is least directly linked to blocked arteries.

Prostate Specific Antigen (PSA). Prostate Specific Antigen comes from the prostate. A high PSA can mean cancer is present, but it usually is only associated with infection or non-cancer enlargement.

Treadmill Stress Test. A stress test helps to determine whether chest pain is coming from the heart. The patient walks or runs on a treadmill until their heart has reached a high stress level. They wear an ECG to look at the heart as it works. A cardiologist then interprets the ECG to see if the heart is getting enough blood flow.

Stress ECHO. The patient walks or runs on the treadmill, but instead of just an ECG, an ultrasound is used to look at the shape of the beating heart while it is working. A stress ECHO is more accurate than a plain stress test at finding women's heart disease.

ECHO. This is an ultrasound of the heart that looks at the shape and function of the different chambers and valves. Usually if someone has a heart murmur or heart failure, this is the test that is ordered to get more details.

Holter Monitor. A Holter is an ECG that the patient wears for a 24-hour period. If a patient is having irregular heartbeats or palpitations, this test is ordered to look at those beats while they are occurring. This test gives very accurate information. However, the patient should be having the unusual sensation every day before this test is ordered.

Handheld Event Recorder. An event recorder is a smaller, very portable ECG machine. It does not get as much reliable information as the Holter. However, it is more convenient, because the patient does not wear the machine all of the time. Then, if unusual heartbeats happen, the patient simply puts the device to their chest and the device records a short run of ECG. Doctors order Event Recorders when a patient is having irregular rhythms less than once a day. The patient usually keeps the machine for about a month, then uses it whenever they need.

Cardiology Procedures

Nuclear Stress Test. Versions of this are also called
Adenosine Stress Test, Dobutamine Stress Test, or MUGA
Nuclear Test. This kind of stress test is ordered for people
who can't walk on a treadmill. A chemical is used to make the
heart beat hard and fast and then a dye is used to measure
blood flow to the heart muscle.

These guidelines are from the Advisory Committee on Immunization Practices, updated July 2004. Each vaccine has particular indications and risks and the final determination can only be made with the help of your doctor.

Flu. Influenza. Administered once per year in the fall. Flu shots are recommended for nearly every adult.

Hepatitis A. Two doses required six months apart. This shot is for people who travel out of the US. It is also for people with chronic liver disease, or people who are exposed to blood or body fluids, such as IV drug users, patients with clotting factor disorders who might receive transfusions, men who have sex with men, or any individual who has multiple sex partners.

Hepatitis B. All adolescents. (Most common guidelines recommend starting at infancy.) Three doses required over six months for people who are exposed to other people with hepatitis, or who are exposed to blood or body fluids such as IV drug users, patients with clotting factor disorders, men who have sex with men, or anyone with multiple sex partners.

Meningococcal. Two. Routinely recommended for people with higher exposure to meningococcal disease. This includes mostly young adults moving to college.

Pneumonia. There are two:
Prevnar 13 – Give once after 65 yo.
Pneumovax 23 - Usually this is a single dose given after the age of 65. However, if the first dose is given before age 65 then a booster is recommended at 65 years old. It should also be everyone who has a chronic disease such as CHF,, diabetes liver disease, poor immune system, etc, or if they have had their spleen removed.

Immunizations

Tetanus. Td. Administered every ten years. It should be given to all adults at 10-year intervals. Getting an open cut is often the reminder since that is how tetanus is transmitted.

Shingles. Zostavax is recommended for every adult to prevent shingles. It is recommended for everyone at age 60 or anyone over 60 who never received the vaccine. Only one injection is needed and the vaccine lasts a lifetime.

Acute. Indicates that something is temporary, or it could represent an illness or injury that happened very recently – usually on the order of hours or a few days. The opposite of acute is *chronic*.

Benign. Not cancerous. This refers to any lump, mass or tumor that is not a cancer. Whatever it is made of, it will not tend to spread or grow at distant sites. There still might be some local effect. For example, a benign tumor could press on a nerve. And it would not be unusual to have to remove a tumor even if it is benign. In general, benign is good and usually does not lead to long-term problems and rarely would result in death. The opposite of benign is *malignant*.

Congestive Heart Failure (CHF). I never like to use this term because it sounds so... devastating. It does not mean that the heart is going to "fail." It does mean that the heart is not pumping as strongly as it should. There are a number of different things that can result in CHF, including high blood pressure, rheumatic fever, viruses that infect the heart, or just getting older.

Chronic. Signifies that a disease or illness is going to last a long time, maybe even be permanent. The opposite of chronic is *acute*.

Chronic Obstructive Pulmonary Disease (COPD). Emphysema is the older name for this problem. A patient with COPD has stiff lungs that can't move the air into the lungs and then across into the bloodstream.

Malignant. Refers to a cancer. This tumor or bunch of cells can spreads to other places in the body and cause harm, up to death, if not eliminated completely. The opposite of malignant is *benign*.

Palpitations. Means that the patient can feel their heart beating in their chest. Usually this indicates that the heart feels like it is beating too fast or in an irregular way.

Radiology Tests

X-ray. This is the oldest and most common kind of radiology test. X-rays are used to see through the skin and see what is going on with hard structures inside – usually the bones. The most common example is the use of an X-ray to see fractures. Plain X-rays are also good to take at the initial evaluation of the lungs to look for nodules, pneumonia, or heart failure. Abdominal X-rays are used for finding bowel obstruction and kidney stones.

Computed Tomography (CT scan). Often called a "cat" scan, this type of scan uses plain X-rays but gives a two-dimensional picture. There is significantly more radiation with a CT scan, but it provides more detailed information. It is possible to clarify nodules in the lungs, abdominal masses such as liver or pancreas changes, or to look at the appendix. CT scans are often the first test used to look at the brain. Bleeding or old strokes can be seen here. In the brain, CT scans do not show as much detail as a MRI, but are less expensive and more comfortable. Getting a CT scan takes about 30 minutes, and the machine is large and open.

Mammogram. Most people know that a mammogram is used to screen for breast cancer. This form of X-ray test looks for tiny calcium deposits. Mammography is actually not quite as good at telling what a "lump" is made of, so if something is noticed during a breast exam and the doctor wants to know what it is, an ultrasound of the breast is ordered.

Ultrasound. An ultrasound uses sound waves to look inside the body. There is no radiation exposure during this test, which is nice. Ultrasounds are good at identifying differences between soft tissue, such as showing the difference between fluid and solid tissue, in a breast lump. (Fluid means the lump is a cyst and that is a good finding.) Ultrasounds are also good at finding gallstones, kidney stones, or an inflamed appendix, or at looking at bumps in the arms or legs that can not otherwise be identified.

Doppler. This is a fancy ultrasound that can also see the movement of fluid. Doppler is basically used to look at blood flow, such as identifying blockage in the carotid arteries in the neck, or a blood clot in the leg.

ECHO. This is a Doppler test of the heart. Usually these are done by a cardiologist's office.

Magnetic resonance imaging (MRI). This is one of the most expensive and time-consuming tests available today. The good news is that there is no radiation with a MRI. The bad news it that to get the test, the patient has to lay very still, for 30 to 60 minutes, in a machine that is very narrow and makes a lot of noise. Some people who are claustrophobic do not tolerate MRI tests. We order a MRI to see specific little details - such as a small stroke or tumor in the brain. MRI tests are also commonly used to see inside joints - such as the meniscus or ligaments in the knee, or to look at the nerves, discs, and bones of the spine.

DEXA. Bone density test sometimes incorrectly called a bone scan. This test uses X-rays to measure the density of bones. We order a DEXA scan to determine if someone has osteoporosis.

Nuclear Bone Scan. This kind of test is usually done in a hospital. The patient is given a dose of radioactive "tracer" that goes to a specific location. The machine then measures where that tracer is located and can tell if there is something abnormal about a certain body part. Subtle broken bones or thyroid nodules are some of the reasons nuclear bone scans are ordered.

Screening and Prevention

A screening test is a blood test, exam or procedure that discovers a disease before the patient has any symptoms. To be useful, a screening test is also able to discover the disease early enough to do something about it before it causes significant illness or death. The list that follows is my own opinion. I try to follow recommendations published by the American Academy of Family Physicians, and the U. S. Preventive Services Task Force. I included both tests that are recommended, and some that are not and gave an explanation. Also the recommendations change over time. And of course, based on particular circumstances and the opinion of your physician, screening guidelines might be different. As in the rest of this book, the purpose is to educate and encourage conversation, not be authoritative.

In my own office, I usually think of screening tests when people ask for a physical. If someone has a specific symptom or problem, then that is a different situation. That is NOT screening and what follows has nothing to do with that situation. I also included in this section the preventive recommendation regarding aspirin, because I think to remind people when we are talking about other "healthy" stuff.

Aspirin. Using aspirin is recommended to prevent heart disease and stroke. The exact dose has not been determined, but anywhere from 81 mg to 325 mg is suggested. The risks of taking an aspirin are rare, but include internal bleeding or developing an ulcer.

Breast cancer and mammograms. All women aged 40 years and older should receive a mammogram every one to two years. The largest benefit is for women between the ages of 50 and 70 years old. If a woman is older than 70, she should continue to receive mammograms as long as she is healthy. There is no significant risk from a mammogram.

144

Carotid Artery Doppler. This test checks for blockage of the arteries in the neck. There have been suggestions that people should have this test to prevent strokes. Unfortunately, getting a Doppler test in people who have not had a stroke or TIA actually has not been show to prevent strokes. That is because the treatment, surgery, can actually lead to someone having a stroke. Therefore, currently I do not recommend that people with no symptoms get this test. However, this is an area of medicine that is changing. There are ongoing technological advances that make newer treatments, such as stints, less risky. Therefore, these guidelines will probably change. Also, despite the fact that the screening guidelines don't support everyone doing this test, there are many commercial companies that offer Doppler for a reasonable fee. If you want to pay for it yourself, the information might add value and any information you obtain you should relay to your doctor.

Colon Cancer Screening. Colonoscopy. Hemoccult cards. All adults should have screening for colon cancer beginning at age 50 years. Colonoscopy, occult blood (otherwise known as stool cards), barium enema and sigmoidoscopy are all helpful. The frequency of testing ranges from once per year to every ten years, and depends on the kind of test and other patient factors. Therefore the guidelines leave the choice of test and timing up to the patient and their doctor. CT with contrast, sometimes called virtual colonoscopy has NOT been proven to be helpful and therefore is NOT recommended.

Dementia. Current recommendations are to NOT screen for dementia. People often see information in the lay press about genetic tests. None of these are readily available. Further, even if they were available, it is impossible to predict who would develop a severe case and a mild care.

Screening and Prevention

Depression. It is good to screen for depression in all adults, if it takes place in a setting in which treatment is available. There is no suggested interval or particular test. There are a number of different questions that can be asked or forms a patient can fill out to find depression.

Diabetes. It is NOT necessary to screen for diabetes. Because people with diabetes take many years to occur, there is no advantage to finding the disease in its "early" stages.

Heart disease. People, who have low or normal risk, should NOT be tested with EKGs, treadmill tests, "calcium scores" or CT scan. There are however a number of risk factors including male sex, age, family history, smoking, high blood pressure, diabetes, obesity, sedentary life style, and high cholesterol which might be taken into account and make one of the tests appropriate for certain individuals. Based on some of these factors, the patient and their doctor could consider doing an evaluation.

Hepatitis. The current guidelines say we should NOT screen for hepatitis.

Lung cancer. Screening for lung cancer using chest x-ray, CT scan, sputum tests, and combinations of all of these is controversial. The panel could not recommend either for or against the use of these tests. There is risk from radiation exposure. There is also a risk of getting a false positive test and then performing a procedure that could cause harm to the patient. Therefore the patient and their doctor should decide when one of these tests might be of benefit.

Obesity. It is recommended that all adult patients are screened for obesity and that they should be offered intensive counseling and behavioral interventions to promote sustained weight loss.

Osteoporosis. It is recommended that all women age 65 and older is screened for osteoporosis with a DEXA. No guidelines are listed for the interval of screening. However, at least two years between tests is thought to be accurate since changes occur slowly.

Prostate cancer. PSA. Digital Rectal Exam (DRE). There is not enough evidence regarding prostate cancer screening to recommend for or against this test. These guidelines apply to both the PSA blood test and the rectal exam. These recommendations include the evidence that PSA and DRE can find prostate cancer at an earlier stage, but there are a number of harmful interventions that might occur from a false positive. These include anxiety, biopsies, and potential adverse effects of treatments resulting from an incorrect diagnosis.

Web Sites

I have listed some common websites that I recommend for patients. And there is plenty of space to add your favorites.

www.aafp.org   Academy of Family Physicians

www.aap.org   Academy of Pediatrics

www.mayoclinic.com   Mayo Clinic – general info

www.americanheart.org   American Heart Association

www.cdc.gov   Travel and Immunizations

web site   information

____
____
____
____
____
____
____
____
____
____
____
____
____
____
____
____
____